Contents

What is Abs Diet? 7

What You Need to Know 8

How does Abs Diet work? 10

Will Abs Diet help you lose weight?...............11

Is Abs Diet a heart-healthy diet? 14

Can Abs Diet prevent or control diabetes? 15

Recommended Timing...................16

Exercise Plan 17

Modifications.................................19

What Can You Eat? 20

"Power Foods" 22

"Cheat Meals"...........................24

Smoothies 25

Alcohol 25

Benefits and Drawbacks 25

Potential Health Benefits 29

Potential Health Risks 30

Exercises for defining the abs..................... 32

   Toe reach 34

   Bicycle crunches.............................. 35

   Plank hold.................................... 36

The Best Ways to Get 6-Pack Abs Fast 37

   1. Do More Cardio............................ 38

   2. Exercise Your Abdominal Muscles 40

   3. Increase Your Protein Intake 41

   4. Try High-Intensity Interval Training........ 43

   5. Stay Hydrated 44

   6. Stop Eating Processed Food.................. 46

   7. Cut Back on Refined Carbs 47

8. Fill up on Fiber..............................49

Abs Diet Food List.............................50

Abs Diet Sample Meal Plan 52

Phase 1 (Weeks 1-2)...........................53

Phase 2 (Weeks 3-4)...........................56

Phase 3 (Weeks 5-6)...........................58

Phase 4 (Weeks 7-8)...........................60

ABS DIET RECIPES 62

Mas Macho Meatballs 62

Eggs Beneficial Sandwich 64

The I-Am-Not-Eating-Salad Salad..................66

Bodacious Brazilian Chicken 68

Strawberry Field Marshall Smoothie 71

Guac and Roll....................................72

Chile-Peppered Steak...........................73

Guilt-Free BLT 75

Philadelphia Fryers 76

Banana Split Smoothie 78

Hot Tuna 80

Chili Con Turkey (number of Powerfoods: 4) ... 82

Berry Smoothie 84

Sandwich...................................... 85

BBQ King...................................... 86

Green Eggs and Ham Omelet 89

The Ultimate Power Breakfast 90

Halle Berries Smoothie 92

Guiltless Tailgate Wings...................... 93

Romaines of the Day.......................... 95

The Official Abs Diet Burger 97

Three Amigos Chili........................... 100

The Pesto Resistance 102

Pita Egg Sandwich with Veggies and Cheese . 104

Cinnamon Berry-Nut Oatmeal 107

Chicken and pine nut salad 108

Chicken Guac Sandwich with Tomato, Lettuce

and Onion.. 110

Spicy guacamole chicken.......................... 111

Garlicky dill salmon.................................. 113

Savory Breakfast Pizza 115

Protein Berry Smoothie Bowl..................... 119

LOW CARB CHOCOLATE PROTEIN PANCAKES

RECIPE... 121

What is Abs Diet?

The Abs Diet is a diet and exercise plan that promises a flatter and stronger midsection in six weeks. The Abs Diet is a six-week plan. You eat six times a day and don't count calories, because portion control is built into the program. Dieters alternate larger meals with small snacks; typically you'll have a snack two hours before lunch, another one two hours before dinner and one more two hours after dinner. Each meal must contain at least two of the 12 Abs Diet "Powerfoods," such as almonds, beans, spinach, instant oatmeal, eggs, peanut butter, raspberries, olive oil and whole grains. These are the building blocks of Abs Diet, which was created by David Zinczenko, the former editor in chief of Men's Health. Ample meal plans and recipes are provided, all emphasizing protein, fiber, calcium and healthy fats. Refined carbs, saturated and trans fats, and high-fructose corn syrup are discouraged. You get a "cheat meal" once a week, when you can forget the diet and chow down on whatever you're craving. Exercise is as important as nutrition in the Abs Diet.

What You Need to Know

Despite the lack of restrictions, there are a few guidelines to follow such as portion control, which is strongly encouraged. Zinczenko writes that men commonly eat up to twice as much food as they think they're eating, especially when they consume grains, fats, and sweets. (By contrast, a study conducted by the U.S. Department of Agriculture (USDA) published the same year as "The Abs Diet" found that food recall in men is generally accurate.)

To avoid overconsuming food, Zinczenko encourages those who follow the diet to watch portion sizes of all foods, but especially those containing fat (such as peanut butter) or carbohydrates like rice, bread, and pasta. The diet recommends consuming no more than 1–2 servings per food group at each meal. He also advises that the total contents of your meal should fit on one dinner plate without piling the food too high.

Making certain key food choices is also important on this plan. You are encouraged to eat "energy-efficient foods." In general, these are foods that are nutrient-dense—meaning that they provide more macronutrients, vitamins, and minerals for fewer calories. For example, beans are encouraged. Kidney beans, black beans, pinto beans, and others provide fiber and protein and are relatively low in calories when prepared without oil or other fats. Nuts, whole grains, and berry-rich protein smoothies are also emphasized.

How does Abs Diet work?

You'll need to cut out certain foods and emphasize others to get started on the Abs Diet. Here are some tips:

• Stop eating sugary cereals, packaged dinners, cookies and crackers

- Add two or three Powerfoods to each of your three major meals

- Include at least one Powerfood into one of your three snacks

- Drink lots of smoothies, which don't take much time to make. Smoothies with Powerfoods such as berries, whey powder and peanut butter satisfy sweet-tooth cravings. Aim for an 8-ounce smoothie for breakfast, as a substitute for a meal, or as a snack before or after a workout

Will Abs Diet help you lose weight?

No research has specifically studied the Abs Diet, but it's based on concepts supported by good evidence. Still, there's controversy as to whether many small meals or fewer large meals is best for weight loss.

- People in a study who ate smaller meals more frequently – four to six times a day – were half as likely to become overweight as were those who ate three or fewer larger meals. Regular snacks and meals help keep blood sugar levels stable and control the release of insulin, a hormone that causes the body to store fat, according to findings published in 2003 in the American Journal of Epidemiology. Eating fewer, larger meals, on the other hand, spikes insulin levels. That's why the Abs Diet calls for a total of six meals and snacks spread evenly throughout the day.

- A tightly controlled 2013 study out of Cornell University, on the other hand, found that skipping one meal a day led to eating about 400 fewer calories that day overall. Other research has supported intermittent fasting as an effective weight loss tool.

- Researchers at Purdue University found that people feel fuller longer when they drink thick drinks (like the Powerfoods smoothies in the Abs Diet) than when they drink thin ones, even when calories, temperatures and amounts are equal. And another study found that women who drank skim milk after exercising lost 3 1/2 pounds in 12 weeks, while a group of women who drank sports drinks gained weight. Abs Diet smoothies typically include 1 percent or skim milk.

- The value of all 12 Powerfoods is supported by research. A 2009 study in the American Journal of Clinical Nutrition, for example, found that eating almonds suppresses hunger, aiding weight loss efforts. Extra-protein whey powder, which can be added to Abs Diet meals and smoothies, is another diet tool. Research suggests that people who eat more protein are more likely to stick to their diets for a year than are those who eat more carbohydrates.

Is Abs Diet a heart-healthy diet?

There isn't a ton of research on Abs Diet. But the program reflects the medical community's widely accepted definition of a heart healthy diet – it's heavy on fruits, veggies and whole grains, and light on saturated and trans fats. Such an approach is considered the best way to keep cholesterol and blood pressure in check and heart disease at bay.

Can Abs Diet prevent or control diabetes?

No research has studied the potential of the Abs Diet to prevent or control diabetes. However, some of the Powerfoods are backed up by studies that suggest they may protect against the disease, and being overweight is a major risk factor for Type 2 diabetes. If the Abs Diet helps you lose weight and keep it off, you'll almost certainly tilt the odds in your favor. In fact, experts generally consider an approach like the Abs Diet's to be the gold standard of diabetes prevention – it emphasizes the right foods, discourages the wrong ones and mandates physical activity.

Recommended Timing

Eating frequency is another key component of the Abs Diet. Followers are advised to eat six meals per day—three relatively small meals and three snacks. Zinczenko claims that eating three large meals creates an hourly energy imbalance that is associated with a fatter body. By eating regularly throughout the day, he claims you are able to keep your energy input (food consumption) and energy output (activity) in balance to maximize fat loss and muscle gain.

Zinczenko also writes that eating more often helps to improve satiety and reduce the risk of binge-eating. Satiety is a feeling of satisfaction and fullness that you are likely to feel after eating, and boosting satiety is believed to help avoid severe hunger that can lead to overeating.

As a specific schedule, the Abs Diet alternates larger meals with smaller snacks. It is recommended that you eat two of your snacks two hours before lunch and dinner, and one snack two hours after dinner. If you eat over the course of a 12-hour day, you can expect to eat about every three hours.

Exercise Plan

The exercise plan is fundamental to the Abs Diet. Followers of the program should expect to exercise at least three times per week for a minimum of 20 minutes per session. The exercise plan has three components:

Strength training performed three times per week. Each session is a total-body workout and one places special emphasis on the legs.

Strength exercises are compiled into a circuit format with little to no rest between exercises. Typical exercises include the military press, upright row, leg extension, biceps curl, and bench press.

- Abdominal exercises are performed two times per week. Ab exercises include the traditional abdominal crunch, bent-leg knee raise, and side bridge.

- Cardiovascular exercise is optional on non-strength-training days. Activities like cycling, running, or swimming are recommended. At least some light cardiovascular activity (like walking) is recommended for at least two of your three off days.

Modifications

Those with dietary restrictions should be able to follow the Abs Diet for the full six weeks. Vegans and vegetarians should be able to eat well on this program, although vegans will need to find an alternative to whey protein powder (such as pea protein powder or soy protein powder) for smoothies. Since whole grains, legumes, fruits, and vegetables are encouraged, plant-based eaters will find plenty to fill their plates at mealtime.

Those who adhere to a gluten-free diet will also be able to follow the program, choosing whole grains like quinoa or buckwheat instead of gluten-containing grains.

What Can You Eat?

The Abs Diet is promoted as a simple-to-follow plan because few foods are restricted, no calorie counting is required, and it allows you to eat frequently throughout the day. Also, there is no strict carbohydrate restriction, which was a key feature of many diets that were popular when "The Abs Diet" was first published. This may have helped to set it apart from other fat loss programs at the time.

The six-week plan encourages whole fruits and vegetables, lean protein sources, whole grains, healthy fats, and whey protein. Smoothies are also a cornerstone of the diet and can take the place of a meal or a snack.

The book provides followers with guidelines about beverages and suggests they avoid alcohol. Beverages that are encouraged include low-fat or fat-free milk, green tea, and diet soda (in moderation). Zinczenko also recommends consuming at least eight glasses of water per day.

What to Eat

- Whole grains

- Lean meat

- Vegetables

- Lowfat dairy

- Beans

- Fruit (especially fiber-rich berries)

- Nuts

- Protein powder

- Any food you desire for a "cheat meal"

What Not to Eat

- Fatty meat

- Refined grains

- Alcoholic beverages

- Sweetened cereals

- Cookies, candy, processed sweet treats

- Processed microwavable meals

- Other foods containing trans fat or high fructose corn syrup

"Power Foods"

As a key part of the program, you are required to add at least two "power foods" to each meal and snack that you consume. There are 12 total foods on the list and readers are encouraged to remember the foods because the names align with the concept of the book:

- Almonds and other nuts

- Beans and legumes

- Spinach and other green vegetables

- Dairy (fat-free or low-fat milk, yogurt, cheese)

- Instant oatmeal (unsweetened, unflavored)

- Eggs

- Turkey and other lean meats

- Peanut butter

- Olive oil

- Whole-grain breads and cereals

- Extra-protein (whey) powder

- Raspberries and other berries

"Cheat Meals"

Those who follow this diet are encouraged to have what Zinczenko refers to as a "cheat meal" once a week. On this day, there are no guidelines, no portion control rules, no encouraged or discouraged foods. You simply eat the foods that you have been craving or missing. Zinczenko says that the way to control your cravings is to satisfy them every once in a while. He also says that a high-calorie "cheat day" helps to increase the body's metabolism.3

Smoothies

You are encouraged to build smoothies around the 12 power foods, such as protein powder, berries, yogurt, peanut butter, and other ingredients. Smoothies should measure no more than eight ounces.

Alcohol

Due to the substantial calorie content of alcoholic beverages, Zinczenko advises followers to avoid alcohol during the six-week plan. He also believes there is a tendency to eat more whenever alcohol is consumed.

Benefits and Drawbacks

Benefits

- Encourages consumption of nutrient-rich foods

- Includes foods from all food groups

- Promotes daily physical activity

- Includes specific exercise plan

- Maintenance plan included in books

Drawbacks

- Makes substantial health claims

- Cheat day may promote unhealthy eating behavior

- Frequent eating doesn't work for everyone

The Abs Diet is a relatively healthy eating and exercise program, but it may overpromise in terms of some of the benefits. Review the pros and cons to help inform your decision about trying this plan.

Benefits

- Protein-packed nutrition. Foods that are encouraged on the Abs Diet are not only nutrient-rich but are likely to help to build muscle and reduce hunger. For example, many of the foods on the "power foods" list are good sources of protein. Many also contain healthy fat and fiber so that you don't feel deprived.

- Encourages exercise. Another benefit of this plan is that it includes a specific, evidence-based exercise program that incorporates both strength and cardiovascular training, which may lead to weight loss. Many fat loss programs do not provide a specific exercise prescription.

- Maintenance plan included. "The Abs Diet" book includes a maintenance plan to follow once the six-week diet is complete, which may help to promote long-term weight management.

Drawbacks

• Lacks sufficient evidence. The Abs Diet makes substantial claims about certain health benefits, but there is no research specifically related to this particular diet to support it. For example, Zinczenko says that a six-pack is the "ultimate predictor of your health" and that great abs have powers of seduction.

• Encourages unhealthy eating habits. Zinczenko advises eating whatever you want on your "cheat day," which does not promote a healthy relationship with food and encourages overeating.

- Eating frequency may not work for everyone. There is disagreement among nutrition and wellness experts about whether or not frequent eating can promote weight loss. Current research suggests this may not be the most effective strategy.

Potential Health Benefits

May Promote Weight Loss

The Abs Diet encourages healthy, whole foods and regular exercise, which may very well lead to weight loss. Research has shown that combining exercise and diet is more effective for fat loss than exercise or diet alone and that both strength training and cardio are effective exercise modalities.8

While there is some science to support certain aspects of the Abs Diet such as the aforementioned, there is no research that has specifically investigated this plan. Core strengthening exercises can certainly help develop stronger abdominal muscles, but spot reduction of fat in one area of the body is a weight-loss myth.

Potential Health Risks

Eating More Meals Doesn't Always Work

Eating more frequent, smaller meals may have been a health trend when "The Abs Diet" was first published, but more recent studies have suggested that the opposite approach may be smarter for some if fat loss is your goal.

A large research review on the matter was published in Frontiers in Nutrition in 2015. Researchers examined studies that investigated the relationship between eating frequency, food intake, and weight. Eight out of the 13 studies that reported on food consumption found that increasing eating frequency provided no significant benefit. Eleven out of 17 studies that reported on body measurements found that eating more often had no significant effect on body size.

May Create An Unhealthy Relationship With Food

Since "The Abs Diet" was published, the importance of developing a healthy relationship with food has become a focus in the nutrition community. Programs that include "good" foods or "bad" foods have been questioned as they may have a negative impact on eating behaviors.

"Cheat days" and "cheat meals" are also problematic, as these terms associate food with guilty behavior and imply that "cheating" may cause more harm than good. In fact, some studies have found that those who associate food with guilt are more likely to have unhealthy eating habits.

Exercises for defining the abs

The Department of Health and Human Services recommend that adults perform 150–300 minutes of moderate-intensity exercise or 75–

150 minutes of vigorous-intensity aerobic activity each week.

Additionally, adults should also perform muscle-strengthening activities of moderate or greater intensity involving major muscle groups, such as the abdomen, on 2 or more days a week.

Four major muscles comprise the abdominals:

- the external and internal obliques, which help the torso twist from side to side

- the rectus abdominis, which allows the body to bend forward

- the transverse abdominis, which provide stability and strength to the torso

Building defined abs requires exercises that target each of the four abdominal muscles.

Below are three examples that work to build abdominal muscle:

Toe reach

This exercise is good for building the rectus abdominis.

To perform the toe reach:

1. Lie faceup on the floor with the legs extended into the air at 90 degrees to the body.

2. Lift the arms and point the fingers upward toward the toes.

3. Keep the lower back pressed into the floor and exhale while curling the upper back off the floor and reaching the fingers up toward the toes.

4. Lower back to the start.

5. Perform as many repetitions as possible within 30 seconds.

Bicycle crunches

This exercise is good for building the rectus abdominis and obliques

To perform bicycle crunches:

1. Lie faceup on the floor.

2. Interlace the fingers behind the head and curl the knees up to the chest, keeping the lower back flat on the floor.

3. Twist the torso toward the right side, bringing the left elbow over to the right knee. Extend the left leg straight out at the same time.

4. Repeat the twist to the opposite side, crossing the right elbow over and bringing the left leg in to meet it. Extend the right leg straight out.

5. Repeat as many times as possible within 30 seconds.

Plank hold

This exercise is good for building the transverse abdominis.

To perform the plank hold:

1. Lie facedown on the ground.

2. Push the body up onto the forearms and toes.

3. Focus on keeping a straight line from the shoulders to the heels. Do not let the back arch or sag toward the ground.

4. Hold for 30 seconds, then rest.

People can also perform a side plank variant, which is another exercise to work the obliques.

Cardiovascular exercise, such as running, dancing, and swimming, is also important to reduce overall body fat. High intensity interval training (HIIT) can be particularly impressiveTrusted Source at burning fat.

The Best Ways to Get 6-Pack Abs Fast

Whether you're aiming to achieve your fitness goals or simply want to look good in a swimsuit, acquiring a sculpted set of six-pack abs is a goal shared by many.

Getting a six-pack requires dedication and hard work, but you don't have to hit the gym seven days a week or become a professional bodybuilder to do so.

Instead, a few modifications to your diet and lifestyle can be enough to produce serious, long-lasting results.

Here are 8 simple ways to achieve six-pack abs quickly and safely.

1. Do More Cardio

Cardio, also called aerobic exercise, is any form of exercise that increases your heart rate.

Regularly incorporating cardio into your routine can help you burn extra fat and speed your way to a set of six-pack abs.

Studies show that cardio is especially effective when it comes to reducing belly fat, which can help make your abdominal muscles more visible.

One small study showed that doing cardio exercise three to four times per week significantly decreased belly fat in 17 men.

Another review of 16 studies found that the more cardio exercise people did, the greater amount of belly fat they lost.

Try to get in at least 20–40 minutes of moderate to vigorous activity per day, or between 150–300 minutes per week.

Activities like running, walking, biking, swimming or engaging in your favorite sports are just a few easy ways to fit cardio into your day.

2. Exercise Your Abdominal Muscles

The rectus abdominis is the long muscle that extends vertically along the length of your abdomen.

Although most well-known as the muscle that creates the appearance of the six-pack, it's also necessary for breathing, coughing and bowel movements.

Other abdominal muscles include the internal and external obliques and the transverse abdominis.

Exercising these muscles is key to increasing muscle mass and achieving six-pack abs.

However, keep in mind that abdominal exercises alone are unlikely to decrease belly fat.

For example, one study found that doing abdominal exercises five days per week for six weeks had no effect on belly fat in 24 women.

Instead, be sure to pair your abdominal exercises with a healthy diet and regular cardio to boost fat burning and maximize results.

Abdominal crunches, bridges and planks are a few of the most popular exercises that can help strengthen your abdominal muscles and create the appearance of six-pack abs.

3. Increase Your Protein Intake

Upping your intake of high-protein foods can help promote weight loss, fight belly fat and support muscle growth on your road to six-pack abs.

According to one study, consuming high-protein meals helped increase feelings of fullness and promote appetite control in 27 overweight and obese men.

Another study showed that people who increased protein intake by just 15% decreased their calorie intake and saw significant decreases in body weight and body fat.

Consuming protein after working out can also help repair and rebuild muscle tissues as well as aid in muscle recovery.

Plus, one study even found that a high-protein diet helped preserve both metabolism and muscle mass during weight loss.

Meat, poultry, eggs, seafood, dairy products, legumes, nuts and seeds are just a few examples of healthy, high-protein foods that you can add to your diet.

4. Try High-Intensity Interval Training

High-intensity interval training, or HIIT, is a form of exercise that involves alternating between intense bursts of activity and short recovery periods. HIIT keeps your heart rate up and increases fat burning.

Adding HIIT into your routine can boost weight loss and make it even easier to get six-pack abs.

One study showed that young men who performed HIIT training for 20 minutes three times per week lost an average of 4.4 pounds (2 kg) and saw a 17% decrease in belly fat over a 12-week period.

Similarly, another study found that 17 women who did HIIT twice per week for 16 weeks had an 8% decrease in total belly fat.

One of the simplest ways to try HIIT at home is to switch between walking and sprinting for 20–30 seconds at a time.

You can also try alternating between high-intensity exercises like jumping jacks, mountain climbers and burpees with a short break in between.

5. Stay Hydrated

Water is absolutely crucial to just about every aspect of health. It plays a role in everything from waste removal to temperature regulation.

Staying well-hydrated may also help bump up your metabolism, burn extra belly fat and make it easier to get a set of six-pack abs.

In fact, one study found that drinking 500 milliliters of water temporarily increased energy expenditure by 24% for up to 60 minutes after eating.

Other research shows that drinking water may also reduce your appetite and increase weight loss.

One study with 48 middle-aged and older adults found that people who drank water before each meal lost 44% more weight over a 12-week period than those who didn't.

Water requirements can vary based on a variety of factors, including age, body weight and activity level.

However, most research recommends drinking around 1–2 liters (34–68 ounces) of water per day to stay well-hydrated.

6. Stop Eating Processed Food

Heavily processed foods like chips, cookies, crackers and convenience foods are typically high in calories, carbs, fat and sodium.

Not only that, these foods are typically low in key nutrients such as fiber, protein, vitamins and minerals.

Nixing these unhealthy junk foods from your diet and swapping them for whole foods can increase weight loss, reduce belly fat and help you achieve a set of six-pack abs.

This is because it takes more energy to digest whole foods rich in protein and fiber, which can burn more calories and keep your metabolism up.

The nutrients in whole foods, like protein and fiber, also keep you feeling fuller to curb cravings and aid in weight loss.

Fruits, vegetables, whole grains and legumes are all nutritious alternatives to prepackaged convenience items like frozen meals, baked goods and salty snacks.

7. Cut Back on Refined Carbs

Cutting back on your consumption of refined carbohydrates can help you lose extra fat and gain six-pack abs.

Refined carbs lose most of their vitamins, minerals and fiber during processing, resulting in a final product that is low in nutritional value.

Eating lots of refined carbs can cause spikes and crashes in blood sugar levels, which can lead to increased hunger and food intake.

Eating plenty of whole grains, on the other hand, has been linked to a reduced waist circumference and lower body weight.

In fact, one study found that people who ate a high amount of refined grains tended to have a higher amount of belly fat compared to those who ate more whole grains.

Swap out refined carbs from foods like pastries, pastas and processed foods and instead enjoy whole grains such as brown rice, barley, bulgur and couscous to help support satiety and burn belly fat.

8. Fill up on Fiber

Adding more high-fiber foods into your diet is one of the simplest methods for increasing weight loss and achieving six-pack abs.

Soluble fiber moves through the gastrointestinal tract undigested and can help slow the emptying of the stomach to make you feel fuller for longer.

In fact, one review found that increasing fiber intake by 14 grams per day was linked to a 10% decrease in calorie intake and 4.2 pounds (1.9 kg) of weight loss.

Research shows that getting enough fiber in your diet may also prevent weight gain and fat accumulation.

One study showed that for each 10-gram increase of soluble fiber taken daily, participants lost 3.7% of belly fat over five years without making any other modifications in terms of diet or exercise.

Fruits, vegetables, whole grains, nuts and seeds are just a few healthy, high-fiber foods that you can add to your diet to help burn belly fat.

Abs Diet Food List

The Abs Diet eliminates processed foods and added sugar and other unhealthy foods and includes a wide variety of nutrient-dense, whole foods that you can eat. The following shopping list provides suggestions to help you get started on the six-week plan. Note that this is not a definitive shopping list and there may be other foods that you prefer.

- Dark leafy greens (kale, spinach, bok choy, arugula, lettuces)

- Bright-colored vegetables (broccoli, eggplant, bell peppers, beets, tomatoes)

- Fruit (blueberries, blackberries, strawberries, grapefruit, cherries, pineapple)

- Lean meat and fish (chicken and turkey breast, lean ground beef, salmon, tuna)

- Whole grains (brown rice, oats, quinoa)

- Legumes (black beans, pinto beans, chickpeas, lentils)

- Nuts and seeds (almonds, walnuts, cashews, chia seeds, flaxseeds)

- Low-fat dairy products

- Avocados

- Olive oil

- Eggs

- Whey protein powder

Abs Diet Sample Meal Plan

"The Abs Diet" book features a variety of compliant recipes for meals and specialty smoothies like the Abs Diet Ultimate Power Smoothie, the Banana Split Smoothie, and the

Halle Berries Smoothie.3 The protocol outlined in the book includes sample meal plans for those in need of extra guidance.   '

The following three-day meal plan offers additional suggestions for getting started on the Abs Diet. Note that this meal plan is not all-inclusive, and if you do choose to follow this program there may be other meals that you prefer. Just be sure to remember to eat three meals and three snacks and include a smoothie every day.

Phase 1 (Weeks 1-2)

Breakfast

- 4 egg whites

- 1 whole egg

- 3 oz chicken breast

- ½ cup green pepper

- 1 medium apple

Snack

- Coconut-Lime Chicken Bites with Baked Zucchini Fries

Lunch

- 4 oz turkey breast, boneless, skinless

- ½ cup brown cooked rice

- 1 cup broccoli, steamed

- ½ large grapefruit

Snack

- ⅔ cup cottage cheese

- ¼ cup blueberries

- 10 almonds, chopped

Dinner

- Spicy Citrus Shrimp with Quinoa

Bedtime

- 20g whey protein isolate

- ½ tbsp peanut butter, natural

Daily Totals:

- Calories: 1,480

- Protein: 169g

- Carbs: 119g

- Fat: 40g

Phase 2 (Weeks 3-4)

Breakfast

- 3 oz chicken breast, boneless, skinless

- 3 egg whites

- 1 whole egg

- ½ cup green pepper

- 6 almonds (as a side)

Snack

- Purple Sweet Potato Parfait

Lunch

- 4 oz turkey breast, boneless, skinless

- ½ cup brown cooked rice

- 1 cup broccoli, steamed

- ½ large grapefruit

Snack

- ⅔ cup cottage cheese

- ¼ cup blueberries

- 10 almonds, chopped

Dinner

- Chicken Kabobs with Mediterranean Brown

Bedtime

- 20g whey protein isolate

- ½ tbsp peanut butter, natural

Daily Totals:

- Calories: 1,437

- Protein: 164g

- Carbs: 124g,

- Fat: 34g

Phase 3 (Weeks 5-6)

Breakfast

- ½ cup oatmeal, uncooked

- 20g chocolate whey protein

- ½ tbsp coconut oil

Snack

- ½ cup egg whites

- 3 oz chicken breast, boneless, skinless

- ½ cup green peppers, chopped

- ½ large grapefruit

Lunch

- 1 cup broccoli

- ½ cup cooked brown rice

- 4 oz turkey breast, boneless, skinless

Snack

- Baked Sole with Grapefruit Avocado Salsa and ½ cup brown rice

Dinner

- Sweet Chili-Lime Barbecue Chicken with Cucumber Salad

Bedtime

- 6 egg whites

- 1 cup baby spinach

Daily Totals: 1,311 calories, 152g protein, 122g carbs, 24g fat

Phase 4 (Weeks 7-8)

Breakfast

- ½ cup oatmeal, uncooked

- 20g vanilla whey protein

- 1 tbsp flaxseed

- Dash of cinnamon

Snack

- ½ cup egg whites

- 3 oz chicken breast, boneless, skinless

- 2 oz avocado

- ½ large grapefruit

Lunch

- 1 cup broccoli

- 4 oz cooked sweet potato

- 4 oz turkey breast, boneless, skinless

Snack

- Beef Lettuce Wraps

Dinner

- Barbecue Tilapia with Mango Salsa and 1 cup asparagus

Snack

- 6 egg whites

- 1 cup baby spinach

ABS DIET RECIPES

Trying abs-friendly recipes is a great way to explore new flavors and find new favorite dishes while looking after your health. In this part are nourishing abs diet recipes for you to enjoy.

Mas Macho Meatballs

Prepartion time

30 minutes

Ingredients

- 1 pound extra-lean ground beef

- ½ cup crushed saltine crackers

- 1 large onion, diced

- 1 clove garlic, minced

- 1 tablespoon ground flaxseed or whey powder

- 1 jar (16 ounces) tomato sauce

- 4 whole-wheat hoagie rolls

- ½ cup reduced-fat mozzarella cheese, shredded

Ingredients

1. Mix the beef, crackers, onion, garlic, and flaxseed or whey powder into golf ball-size meatballs.

2. In a nonstick skillet over medium heat, cook the meatballs until browned all the way around.

3. Drain the fat from the skillet, and add the tomato sauce.

4. While the mixture is warming, use a fork to scoop out some of the bread in the rolls to form shallow trenches.

5. Spoon the meatballs and sauce into each trench, and sprinkle with shredded mozzarella, and top with the top half of the roll.

Eggs Beneficial Sandwich

Prepartion time

15 minutes

Ingredients

- 1 large whole egg

- 3 large egg whites

- 1 teaspoon ground flaxseed

- 2 slices whole-wheat bread, toasted

- 1 slice Canadian bacon

- 1 tomato, sliced, or 1 green bell pepper, sliced

- ½ cup orange juice

Ingredients

1. Scramble the whole egg and egg whites in a bowl.

2. Add ground flaxseed to the mixture.

3. Fry in a nonstick skillet spritzed with vegetable oil spray, and dump onto the toast.

4. Add bacon and tomatoes, peppers, or other vegetables of your choice.

The I-Am-Not-Eating-Salad Salad

Prepartion time

10 minutes

Ingredients

- 2 ounces grilled chicken

- 1 cup romaine lettuce

- 1 tomato, chopped

- 1 small green bell pepper, chopped

- 1 medium carrot, chopped

- 3 tablespoons Italian 94% fat-free Italian dressing or

- 1 teaspoon of olive oil

- 1 tablespoon grated Parmesan cheese

- 1 tablespoon ground flaxseed

Ingredients

1. Chop the chicken into small pieces.

2. Mix all the ingredients together, and store in the fridge.

3. Eat on multigrain bread or by itself.

Bodacious Brazilian Chicken

Prepartion time

30 minutes

Ingredients

- 1 lemon

- 1 lime

- 1 tablespoon ground flaxseed

- 1 can (8 ounces) tomato sauce

- 1 can (6 ounces) frozen orange juice concentrate

- 1½ cloves garlic, minced

- 1 teaspoon dried Italian seasoning

- 4 boneless, skinless chicken breast halves

- 1 teaspoon hot pepper salsa

- ½ cup chunky salsa

Ingredients

1. Grate the zest of the lemon and lime into a resealable bag.

2. Squeeze the juice from both fruits into the bag, and throw out the pulp and the seeds.

3. Mix in everything else except the chicken and salsa.

4. Drop in the chicken, reseal the bag, and refrigrate for a few hours.

5. Grill the chicken, turning and basting with marinade a few times, for 10 to 15 minutes or until the center is no longer pink.

6. Serve with salsa.

Strawberry Field Marshall Smoothie

Prepartion time

10 minutes

Ingredients

- ½ cup low-fat vanilla yogurt

- 1 cup 1% milk

- 2 teaspoons peanut butter

- 1 cup frozen strawberries

- 2 teaspoons whey powder

- 6 ice cubes, crushed

Instructions

1. Blend all ingredients together.

Guac and Roll

Prepartion time

15 minutes

Ingredients

- 1 can (6 ounces) light oil-packed tuna

- 2/3 cup guacamole

- ¼ cup chopped tomatoes

- 1 teaspoon lemon juice

- 1 tablespoon light mayonnaise

- 1 teaspoon ground flaxseed

- 2 6-inch whole-wheat hoagie rolls

Ingredients

1. Combine the first six ingredients in a bowl and blend thoroughly with a fork.

2. Split the rolls in half, and fill each half with ¼ cup of the mixture.

Chile-Peppered Steak

Prepartion time

30 minutes

Ingredients

- 2 carrots, sliced

- 1 cup chopped broccoli

- 2 jalapeño peppers, sliced

- 2 cayenne peppers, sliced

- 12 ounces lean sirloin steak, sliced thin

- ¼ cup Hunan stir-fry sauce

- 4 cups cooked brown rice

Instructions

1. Heat the oil in a nonstick skillet over high heat.

2. Toss in the carrots and broccoli, and cook until tender.

3. Add the peppers and beef, and continue cooking until meat is done.

4. Add sauce, and serve over rice.

Guilt-Free BLT

Prepartion time

15 minutes

Ingredients

- ¾ tablespoon fat-free mayonnaise

- 1 whole-wheat tortilla

- 2 slices turkey bacon, cooked

- 2 ounces roasted turkey breast, diced

- 2 slices tomato

- 2 leaves lettuce

Instructions

1. Smear the mayo on the tortilla.

2. Line the middle of the tortilla with the bacon and top with turkey breast, tomato, and lettuce.

3. Roll it tightly into a tube.

Philadelphia Fryers

Prepartion time

15 minutes

Ingredients

- 1 medium onion, sliced

- 1 small red bell pepper, sliced

- 1 small green bell pepper, sliced

- 2/3 cup medium or hot salsa

- 4 multigrain hoagie rolls

- ¾ pound roast beef, thinly sliced

- ½ cup grated reduced-fat Cheddar cheese

Instructions

1. In a nonstick skillet over medium heat, cook the onion and peppers until tender.

2. Add the salsa and heat until warm.

3. Construct the sandwiches with the buns, roast beef, onions, peppers, and cheese, then warm them in the microwave for 1 to 2 minutes on high, until the cheese starts to melt.

Banana Split Smoothie

Prepartion time

5 minutes

Ingredients

- 1 banana

- ½ cup low-fat vanilla yogurt

- 1/8 cup frozen orange juice concentrate

- ½ cup 1% milk

- 2 teaspoons whey powder

- 6 ice cubes, crushed

Instructions

1. Blend all ingredients together.

Hot Tuna

Prepartion time

20 minutes

Ingredients

- ½ cup chopped celery

- 1 onion, chopped

- ½ cup shredded, reduced-fat mozzarella cheese

- ½ cup reduced-fat cottage cheese

- 1 can (6 ounces) water-packed tuna, drained and flaked

- ¼ cup reduced-fat mayonnaise

- 1 tablespoon lemon juice

- 3 whole-wheat English muffins, split in half

Instructions

1. Preheat your oven to 350°F. In a large nonstick skillet over low heat, cook the celery and onion until softened.

2. Add the cheeses, tuna, mayo, and lemon juice to the skillet, and cook the mixture just long enough to warm it up.

3. Spread one-sixth of the mixture on each English muffin half.

4. Put the muffin halves on a baking sheet, and bake for 10 minutes.

Chili Con Turkey (number of Powerfoods: 4)

Prepartion time

13 minutes

Ingredients

- 1 pound ground turkey

- 1 can (14 ounces) Mexican-style diced tomatoes

- 1 can (15 ounces) black beans, rinsed and drained

- 1 can (14 ounces) whole-kernel sweet corn, drained

- 1 package (1 ½ ounces) dried chili mix

- 1 tablespoon ground flaxseed

- ¼ cup water

- 1 cup cooked rice

Instructions

1. In a large nonstick skillet over medium-high heat, brown the turkey.

2. Add everything else but the rice, and cook over low heat for 10 minutes.

3. Serve over rice.

Berry Smoothie

Prepartion time

5 minutes

Ingredients

- ¾ cup instant oatmeal, nuked in water or fat-free milk

- ¾ cup fat-free milk

- ¾ cup mixed frozen blueberries, strawberries, and raspberries

- 2 teaspoons whey powder

- 3 ice cubes, crushed

Instructions

1. Blend all ingredients together

Sandwich

Prepartion time

15 minutes

Ingredients

- 1 ½ teaspoons low-fat cream cheese

- 1 whole-wheat pita, halved to make 2 pockets

- 2 slices turkey or ham

- Lettuce or green vegetable

Instructions

1. Spread cream cheese in the pockets of the pita.

2. Stuff with meat and vegetables.

3. Put in mouth.

4. Chew and swallow.

BBQ King

Prepartion time

40 minutes

Ingredients

- 1 small onion, chopped

- 1 can (3 ounces) sliced mushrooms

- 1 clove garlic, minced

- 1 can (16 ounces) baked beans

- 1 can (8 ounces) navy beans, drained

- 1 can (14 ½ ounces) puréed tomatoes

- ¼ cup seasoned bread crumbs

- ¾ tablespoon ground flaxseed

- ¾ tablespoon olive oil

Instructions

1. Preheat your oven to 350°F.

2. Put the kielbasa in a 2-quart baking dish, and bake until browned (about 5 minutes).

3. Drain the fat and set the dish aside.

4. In a nonstick skillet over medium-high heat, cook the onion, mushrooms, and garlic for 5 to 7 minutes.

5. Transfer to the baking dish, then add the beans and tomatoes, plus salt and pepper to taste.

6. Bake for 20 minutes or until the edges bubble.

7. In a small bowl, mix the bread crumbs and flaxseed with the oil.

8. Sprinkle over the sausage mixture, and broil 4 to 5 inches from the heat until the top is golden (about 3 minutes).

Green Eggs and Ham Omelet

Prepartion time

10 minutes

Ingredients

- 2 eggs

- 1 slice Canadian bacon, diced

- 1/3 cup torn baby spinach leaves

- 1 Tbs shredded reduced-fat smoked mozzarella
cheese

Instructions

1. Whisk the eggs in a bowl, then stir in the Canadian bacon and spinach.

2. Coat a nonstick skillet with cooking spray.

3. Pour in the eggs, cook over medium heat until set, and flip.

4. Sprinkle with the cheese and fold the omelet in half.

The Ultimate Power Breakfast

Prepartion time

10 minutes

Ingredients

- 1 egg

- 1 cup one percent mild

- 3/4 cup plain instant oatmeal

- 1/2 cup mixed berries

- 1 Tbs chopped pecans or sliced almonds

- 1 tsp vanilla whey protein powder

- 1 tsp ground flaxseed

- 1/2 banana, sliced

- 1 Tbs plain yogurt

Instructions

1. Whisk everything but the banana and yogurt in a microwavable bowl.

2. Microwave for 2 minutes or until set.

3. Let cool for a minute or two.

4. Top with the banana and yogurt.

Halle Berries Smoothie

Prepartion time

5 minutes

Ingredients

• 3/4 cup instant oatmeal nuked in water or fat-free milk

• 3/4 cup fat-free milk

• 3/4 cup frozen blueberries, strawberries, and raspberries

- 2 tsp vanilla whey protein powder

- 3 ice cubes

Instructions

1. Dump the cooked oatmeal, milk, berries, whey powder, and ice into a blender, and puree until drinkable. (For a sweeter smoothie, add honey to taste.)

Guiltless Tailgate Wings

Prepartion time

15 minutes

Ingredients

- 3 Tbs hot sauce

- 2 Tbs low-sodium Worcestershire sauce

- 1 Tbs Honey

- 1/2 Tsp Paprika

- 1 clove garlic, crushed

- 12 boneless, skinless chicken tenders (about 12 ounces)

- 2 Tbs low-fat bleu cheese dressing

Instructions

1. Mix the hot sauce, Worcestershire, honey, paprika, and garlic in a large bowl. (If the honey clumps, nuke the mixture for 10 to 15 seconds and then stir.)

2. Place the chicken and half of the sauce in a large re-sealable bag.

3. Close and shake to coat each piece.

4. Heat a large skillet over medium heat.

5. Remove the chicken from the bag and cook for 1 to 2 minutes on each side; discard any sauce left in the bag.

6. Add the chicken to the bowl with the remaining sauce mixture and toss to coat. Serve with the dressing.

Romaines of the Day

Prepartion time

10 minutes

Ingredients

- 2 cups chopped romaine lettuce hearts

- 1 avocado, pitted, peeled, and chopped into bite-size pieces

- 1 medium tomato, chopped into bite-size pieces

- 1/2 cup canned black beans, rinsed and drained

- 2 Tbs diced scallion

- 1 Tbs chopped cilantro

- 1 Tbs extra-virgin olive oil

- 1/4 Tsp grated lime zest

- 2 Tsp lime juice

- 1/4 Tsp salt

- 1/2 Tsp pepper

Instructions

1. Mix the lettuce, avocado, tomato, beans, scallion, and cilantro in a large bowl.

2. Mix the oil, lime zest and juice, salt, and pepper in a small bowl.

3. Pour over the salad and toss well to coat.

The Official Abs Diet Burger

Prepartion time

20 minutes

Ingredients

- 1 egg

- 1 lb lean ground beef

- 1/2 cup rolled oats

- 1/3 cup diced onion

- 1/2 cup chopped spinach

- 2 Tbs shredded reduced fat Mexican-blend cheese

- Salt and pepper

- Whole wheat burger buns

Instructions

1. Whisk the egg in a large bowl.

2. Add everything else and mix--your hands are the best tools—until well blended. Form into 4 patties.

3. Place the burgers on a grill over medium-high heat.

4. Cook 4 to 6 minutes per side or to your desired level of doneness.

5. Serve on whole wheat burger buns and top with lettuce and tomato slices. If you have any extra burgers, wrap them in plastic and freeze for later.

Three Amigos Chili

Prepartion time

40 minutes

Ingredients

- 1 Tbs extra-virgin olive oil

- 1 small onion, diced

- 1 lb ground turkey breast

- 1 can (14.5 oz) diced tomatoes with jalapeños

- 1 can (10.5 oz) chickpeas, rinsed and drained

- 1 can (10.5 oz) black beans, rinsed, and drained

- 1 can (10.5 oz) kidney beans, rinsed, and drained

- 1 can (14 oz) low-sodium chicken broth

- 1/2 Tsp salt

- 1/2 Tsp ground cumin

- 1/8 Tsp ground cinnamon

- hot sauce

Instructions

1. Heat the oil in a large saucepan over medium-low heat.

2. Add the onion and cook until soft, about 3 to 5 minutes.

3. Add the turkey and cook, breaking up the pieces with a wooden spoon, until browned, about 5 minutes.

4. Add the tomatoes with juice, beans, broth, and spices.

5. Stir and bring to a boil, then reduce the heat and simmer for 20 minutes. Serve with hot sauce.

The Pesto Resistance

Prepartion time

25 minutes

Ingredients

- 4 oz whole wheat spaghetti

- 1 Tbs extra-virgin olive oil

- 1/2 cup chopped walnuts

- 1 clove garlic, crushed

- 2 cups torn baby spinach leaves

- 1 Tsp dried basil

- Salt and pepper

- 2 Tbs shredded part-skim mozzarella cheese

Instructions

1. Cook the spaghetti according to the package directions. Drain.

2. Heat the oil in a large nonstick skillet over medium-low heat.

3. Add the walnuts and cook for 3 to 4 minutes, stirring frequently.

4. Add the garlic, spinach, and basil.

5. Cook for 3 to 5 minutes, stirring frequently.

6. Season with salt and pepper.

7. Add the pasta and toss to coat; sprinkle with the cheese.

Pita Egg Sandwich with Veggies and Cheese

Prepartion time

25 minutes

INGREDIENTS

- 2 Tsp. extra virgin olive oil

- ½ cup Birds Eye Tri Color Pepper & Onion Blend, thawed

- Ground pepper, to taste

- 2 eggs

- 1 slice Borden Natural Pepper Jack Cheese

- 1 Ezekiel 4:9 Whole Grain Pocket Bread, cut in half

- Optional garnish: Salsa, hot sauce or organic ketchup

Instructions

1. In a small nonstick skillet, sauté frozen veggies in oil until tender.

2. Top with fresh pepper, combine and remove the mixture from the skillet.

3. Set aside.

4. Crack the eggs into a bowl and whisk until fully blended.

5. Add eggs to the skillet and cook over a medium flame.

6. Just before the eggs are fully cooked, add the cheese and vegetables.

7. Use a spatula to carefully fold the egg over on itself.

8. Remove from pan, cut widthwise and place the omelet halves inside the two halves of the pocket bread.

9. Top with salsa, hot sauce or organic ketchup.

Cinnamon Berry-Nut Oatmeal

Prepartion time

10 minutes

INGREDIENTS

- 1 packet Quaker Instant Oatmeal, Original

- 1/2 cup hot milk or water

- Handful of raspberries

- 1/4 cup chopped walnuts

- 1 Tsp. cinnamon

Instructions

1. Combine oatmeal and liquid of choice and cook according to package instructions.

2. After the oats have finished cooking, mix in raspberries, walnuts and cinnamon.

Chicken and pine nut salad

Prepartion time

4 minutes

INGREDIENTS

- 3 oz Hormel Natural Choice Oven Roasted Carved Chicken Breast Strips

- 2 cups baby spinach leaves

- ½ orange, peeled and segmented

- 1 tablespoon pine nuts

- 6 grape tomatoes, halved

- 2 Tbsp. olive oil

Instructions

1. Mix all of the ingredients together in a bowl and serve.

Chicken Guac Sandwich with Tomato, Lettuce and Onion

Prepartion time

INGREDIENTS

- 1 tablespoon Wholly Guacamole Avocado Verde Dip

- 1 Arnold Sandwich Thins Flax & Fiber

- 3 oz Applegate Organics Oven Roasted Chicken Breast

- Red onion, sliced, to taste

- Tomato, sliced, to taste

- 2 Romaine lettuce leaves, halved

Instructions

1. Spread guacamole onto the bread.

2. Stack chicken, onion, tomato and lettuce on bead.

3. Sandwich the two halves together.

Spicy guacamole chicken

Prepartion time

15 minutes

INGREDIENTS

- 1 pound skinless chicken breasts

- Chili powder, to taste

- 15 oz Eden Organic Black Beans, no salt added, drained and rinced

- 14 oz Birds Eye Tri Color Pepper & Onion Blend, thawed

- Wholly Guacamole Guacasalsa Dip, to taste

Instructions

1. Sprinkle chili powder onto the chicken and cook on a lightly greased skillet over medium heat, until golden brown, about 5 minutes on each side.

2. Remove chicken from heat, set aside and cover.

3. Add beans and veggies to the skillet and cook until warm.

4. Spoon a dollop of guacamole onto each chicken breast and serve with bean and vegetable medley.

Garlicky dill salmon

Prepartion time

25 minutes

INGREDIENTS

- 1 cup Greek yogurt, plain

- Olive oil, to taste

- Fresh dill, to taste

- 4 SeaPak Salmon Burgers

- 6 cups arugula

- 1 bag, Alexia Oven Reds with Olive Oil, Parmesan & Roasted Garlic

Instructions

1. Combine yogurt, olive oil and fresh dill set aside.

2. Cook burgers according to the box instructions.

3. Meanwhile, cook the Alexia potatoes according to the bag instructions.

4. Serve salmon burger atop a bed of arugula and drizzle a tablespoon or two of sauce onto the salmon and greens.

5. Spoon potatoes onto the plate.

Savory Breakfast Pizza

Prepartion time

50 minutes

Ingredients

- Parchment paper

- Nonstick cooking spray

- 2 cups riced cauliflower

- Cheesecloth

- ½ cup cooked steel-cut oatmeal

- ½ cup egg whites

- ¼ cup grated Parmesan cheese

- 1 Tbsp. dried parsley flakes

- 1 tsp. garlic powder

- ¾ cup reduced-fat (2%) cottage cheese

- 1 cup arugula

- ½ cup sliced mushrooms

- ½ cup cherry tomatoes halved

- 2 large hard-boiled eggs sliced

Instructions

1. Preheat oven to 400° F.

2. Line a baking sheet with parchment paper.

3. Coat with cooking spray.

4. Set aside.

5. Place riced cauliflower in a large microwave-safe bowl

6. Cook in the microwave oven for 5 minutes, remove and stir, then cook again for another 5 minutes.

7. Carefully place cooled cauliflower on cheesecloth and wring out all extra liquid into another bowl.

8. Discard liquid.

9. Combine cauliflower, oatmeal, egg whites, Parmesan cheese, parsley, and garlic powder in

a large bowl; mix well until thoroughly combined.

10. Form cauliflower mixture into 2 balls, 1 cup each, and place on prepared pan.

11. Flatten gently with hands to form a circular crust.

12. Bake for 20 to 25 minutes, or until crust is firm and golden.

13. When crusts are done, divide cottage cheese equally between crusts.

14. Then distribute arugula, mushrooms, and tomatoes evenly on top between two pizza crusts.

15. Raise oven to 500° F, or turn on the top broiler to high.

16. Bake for an additional 5 minutes, or until mushrooms and tomatoes are blistered.

17. Divide sliced eggs evenly between pizzas.

18. Serve immediately.

Protein Berry Smoothie Bowl

Prepartion time

10 minutes

Ingredients

- ¾ cup unsweetened almond milk

- 1 cup ice

- 1 scoop Openfit Plant-Based Nutrition Shake

- ½ cup + 2 Tbsp. blackberries fresh (or frozen)

- ⅓ cup blueberries fresh (or frozen)

- 5 medium strawberries sliced

- 1 Tbsp. raw almonds chopped

- 2 Tbsp. unsweetened shredded coconut

Instructions

1. Place almond milk, ice, and protein powder in blender; cover.

2. Blend until smooth.

3. Place smoothie in a medium bowl.

4. Top with berries, almonds, and coconut; serve immediately.

LOW CARB CHOCOLATE PROTEIN PANCAKES RECIPE

Prepartion time

20 minutes

INGREDIENTS

- 1/2 cup Whey protein powder (or collagen, or egg white protein powder)

- 1/2 cup Wholesome Yum Blanched Almond Flour

- 3 tbsp Cocoa powder

- 3 tbsp Besti Erythritol (or sweetener of choice)

- 1 tsp Baking powder

- 4 large Eggs

- 1/3 cup Unsweetened almond milk

- 2 tbsp Avocado oil (or melted coconut oil)

- 1 tsp Vanilla extract

- 1/8 tsp Sea salt

Instructions

1. Shake all ingredients together in the Whiskware Batter Mixer.

2. Let the batter sit for 5 minutes.

3. Preheat a pan over medium-low heat.

4. Squeeze batter into the pan to form small circles (3 inches in diameter).

5. Cover with a lid and cook for a couple of minutes, until bubbles form on top.

6. Use a very thin turner to carefully flip the pancakes, then cook for a couple of minutes on the other side.

7. Repeat with the remaining batter.

Printed in Great Britain
by Amazon

83772576R00070